REGIONAL FRAMEWORK FOR COMMUNITY IMCI

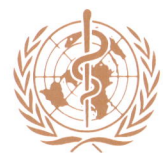

WORLD HEALTH ORGANIZATION
REGIONAL OFFICE FOR THE WESTERN PACIFIC
2003

WHO Library Cataloguing in Publication Data

Regional framework for community IMCI

1. Child health services 2. Disease management 3. Delivery of health care, Integrated

ISBN 92 9061 051 4 (NLM Classification: WA 320)

© World Health Organization 2003

All rights reserved.

The designations employed and the presentation of the material in this publication do not imply the expression of any opinion whatsoever on the part of the World Health Organization concerning the legal status of any country, territory, city or area or of its authorities, or concerning the delimitation of its frontiers or boundaries. Dotted lines on maps represent approximate border lines for which there may not yet be full agreement.

The mention of specific companies or of certain manufacturers' products does not imply that they are endorsed or recommended by the World Health Organization in preference to others of a similar nature that are not mentioned. Errors and omissions excepted, the names of proprietary products are distinguished by initial capital letters.

The World Health Organization does not warrant that the information contained in this publication is complete and correct and shall not be liable for any damages incurred as a result of its use.

Publications of the World Health Organization can be obtained from Marketing and Dissemination, World Health Organization, 20 Avenue Appia, 1211 Geneva 27, Switzerland (tel: +41 22 791 2476; fax: +41 22 791 4857; email: bookorders@who.int). Requests for permission to reproduce WHO publications, in part or in whole, or to translate them – whether for sale or for noncommercial distribution – should be addressed to Publications, at the above address (fax: +41 22 791 4806; email: permissions@who.int). For WHO Western Pacific Regional Publications, request for permission to reproduce should be addressed to Publications Office, World Health Organization, Regional Office for the Western Pacific, P.O. Box 2932, 1000, Manila, Philippines, Fax. No. (632 521-1036, email: publications@wpro.who.int).

TABLE OF CONTENTS

Preface	1
1. Introduction	3
1.1 The IMCI strategy	3
1.2 A brief history of community IMCI	6
1.3 Development of a Western Pacific Regional Framework for Community IMCI	7
2. Overview of the Regional Framework for Community IMCI	8
3. Description of the areas of community IMCI	11
3.1 Partnerships and linkages	11
3.2 Community participation	17
3.3 Health information and promotion	19
3.4 Means for improving key practices	21
4. Links within the Framework and between the three IMCI components	24
4.1 Links between the areas of the framework	24
4.2 Links between the three components of the IMCI strategy	25
5. Roles of different actors in community IMCI implementation	27
6. Guiding principles for community IMCI planning and implementation	31
7. Planning for community IMCI	35
8. Sustainability and scaling-up	38
8.1 Sustainability	38
8.2 Scaling-up	39
9. Monitoring and evaluation	40
Annex 1: Table of planning process	41
Annex 2: Priority indicators for community IMCI	46

PREFACE

The Integrated Management of Childhood Illness (IMCI) strategy was introduced in the Western Pacific Region in 1995. In order to address the unfinished agenda of child survival and to promote the healthy growth and development of children, an increasing number of countries have adopted IMCI as their primary child health strategy.

Composed of three mutually supportive and integrated components, IMCI encompasses interventions both for the health system and for the family and community. While improved health worker skills together with strong health system support for integrated care provide a powerful tool to address common problems in child health services, evidence suggests that improving the way children are treated and cared for in the family and community may potentially have an even greater impact on children's health.

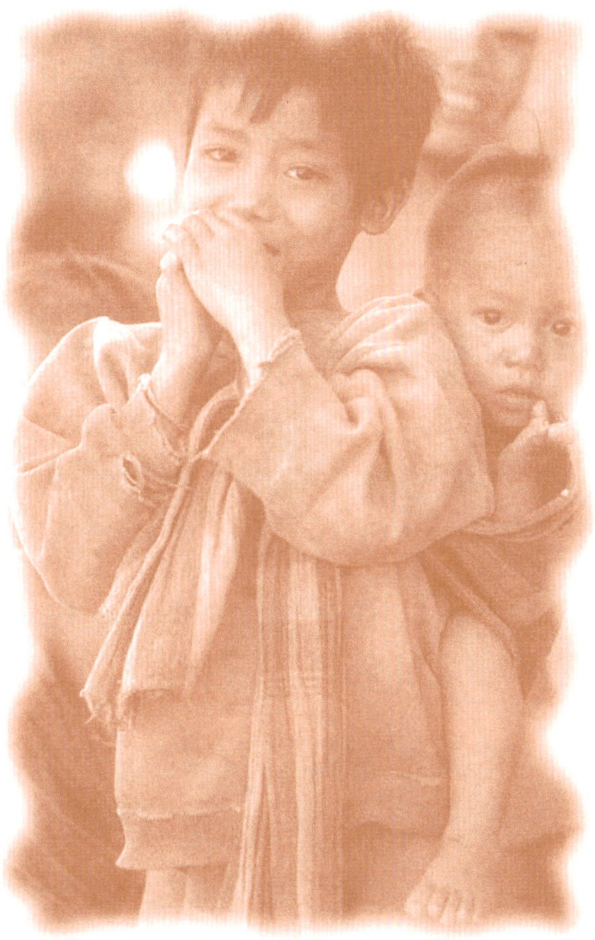

Strengthened family and community action for improved child health can be greatly enhanced by systematic planning for and implementation of community IMCI. Recognizing the complexity of factors that influence child health outcomes, this Regional Framework for Community IMCI has been developed as a practical tool for getting started by building upon existing structures, community actors and actions already in place.

This document is divided into nine chapters. Chapter 1 provides background information about IMCI and describes the context in which this framework was developed. Chapters 2-4 present the Regional Framework for Community IMCI, describe the areas that make up the third component of IMCI, and discuss how the areas are linked to one another and to the other components of IMCI. Chapter 5 details the roles of different actors in community IMCI. Chapter 6 summarizes the guiding principles for community IMCI planning and implementation, and chapter 7 outlines the community IMCI planning process at various levels. Chapter 8 provides suggestions for developing sustainable community-based activities and for scaling-up, and chapter 9 discusses issues related to monitoring and evaluation of community IMCI activities and the need for operations research.

The development of this document has been a consultative process, building upon the experiences of active partners in community child health in the Region. Nevertheless, it is envisioned that the implementation of community IMCI will be a dynamic process, and accumulating experiences from countries will further enrich the Regional Framework. As the importance of partnerships is highlighted throughout the document, I hope that this framework will prove useful for governments and partners alike in working jointly toward a healthy start in life for children in the Western Pacific Region.

Shigeru Omi, MD, Ph.D
Regional Director
WHO Regional Office for the Western Pacific

1. Introduction

1.1 The IMCI strategy

WHO and the United Nations Children's Fund (UNICEF) jointly formulated the IMCI strategy in the mid-1990s in an effort to provide a more integrated approach for addressing the main causes of childhood morbidity and mortality, and for improving child growth and development. IMCI recognizes a child as a whole being, not just as a person with individual illnesses or health problems. The strategy includes elements of prevention as well as curative care. It combines improved management of childhood illness with aspects of nutrition, immunization, disease prevention and health promotion.

The IMCI strategy is made up of the following three components:

1) upgrading the case management and counselling skills of health care providers;
2) strengthening the health system for effective management of childhood illness; and
3) improving family and community practices related to child health and nutrition.

The first two components of IMCI focus on improving the quality of care received by sick children at health facilities. Component 1 requires a local adaptation of standard clinical guidelines and training materials. Once they are adapted, the Ministry of Health and its partners use the materials to train first-level health workers. IMCI can also be

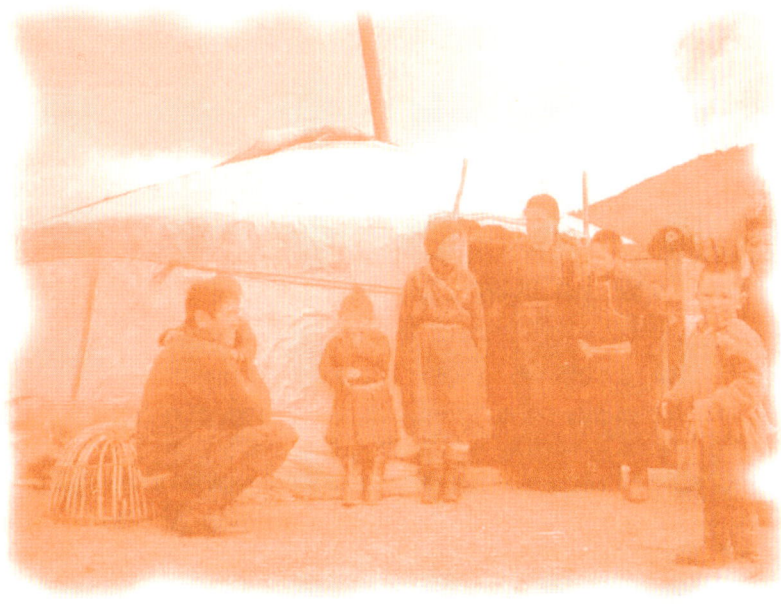

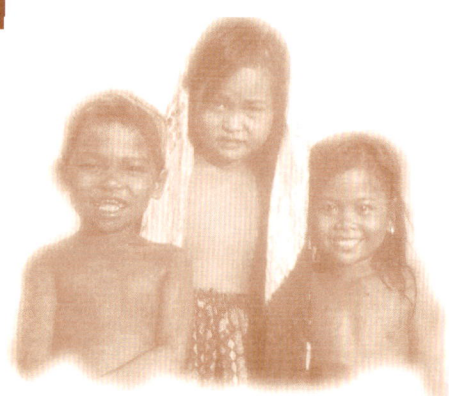

incorporated in the pre-service training curricula of health professionals. For the second component, the Ministry of Health identifies elements of the health system that might make it difficult for health workers to manage childhood illnesses effectively and develops strategies to overcome these elements. Issues that are typically addressed under the second component of IMCI include drug availability, IMCI planning and management, organization of work at health facility level, supervision, referral, health information systems, and health sector reform.

The third component of IMCI focuses on preventive and caring practices at the household and community level. In many countries, there are significant segments of the population that have difficulty accessing basic child health services and interventions. Because many children die from preventable and easily treated illnesses without ever reaching appropriate health services, IMCI works with families and communities to improve their ability to prevent child health problems, to care for both well and sick children, and to make appropriate decisions regarding when and where to seek health care outside the home.

In order to have the greatest impact on child health at the community level, 12 key family practices and four additional areas of importance that contribute to child survival, growth, and development have been identified (see Box 1). Improving key family practices requires the involvement of communities in planning and implementing relevant activities, and can be facilitated by the formation of partnerships between health providers (including traditional healers, private health sector, and agencies with extension services) and communities. Changing behaviours related to the key family practices can be achieved through a number of different programmatic approaches and channels and through the mobilization of the resources of governments, various organizations, and the communities themselves. Typically, a few key family practices are selected initially so as to focus community IMCI efforts and to increase the likelihood of obtaining improved outcomes.

Governments have experience carrying out Components 1 and 2 of the IMCI strategy. Component 3, the community component, has been more of a challenge to implement. This document provides governments with guidance on the implementation of the community component. It also serves as a guide on strategies for implementing activities to promote and strengthen the key family practices in the Western Pacific Region in collaboration with partners.

> ### Box 1. The key family practices
>
> Evidence suggests that families can significantly improve the survival, growth and development of their children by carrying out a limited set of practices. These are:
>
> - Breast-feed infants exclusively for six months. (Mothers found to be HIV positive require counselling about possible alternatives to breast-feeding.)
>
> - Starting at six months of age, feed children freshly prepared energy and nutrient rich complementary foods, while continuing to breast-feed up to two years or longer.
>
> - Ensure that children receive adequate amounts of micronutrients (vitamin A and iron, in particular), either in their diet or through supplementation.
>
> - Dispose of faeces, including children's faeces, safely; and wash hands after defecation, before preparing meals and before feeding children.
>
> - Take children as scheduled to complete a full course of immunizations (BCG, DPT, OPV, and measles) before their first birthday.
>
> - Protect children in malaria-endemic areas, by ensuring that they sleep under insecticide-treated bednets.
>
> - Promote mental and social development by responding to a child's needs for care, and through talking, playing, and providing a stimulating environment.
>
> - Continue to feed and offer more fluids, including breast milk, to children when they are sick.
>
> - Give sick children appropriate home treatment for infections.
>
> - Recognize when sick children need treatment outside the home and seek care from appropriate providers.
>
> - Follow the health worker's advice about treatment, follow-up and referral.
>
> - Ensure that every pregnant woman has adequate antenatal care. This includes having at least four antenatal visits with an appropriate health care provider, and receiving the recommended doses of the tetanus toxoid vaccination. The mother also needs support from her family and community in seeking care at the time of delivery and during the postpartum and lactation period.
>
> Four areas of critical importance complement these 12 key family practices. Work is ongoing to specify the precise behaviours to be supported for each of the areas:
>
> - Adopt and sustain appropriate behaviour regarding prevention and care for HIV/AIDS affected people, including orphans.
>
> - Take appropriate actions to prevent and manage child injuries and accidents.
>
> - Prevent child abuse and neglect, and take appropriate action when it has occurred.
>
> - Ensure that men actively participate in providing childcare, and are involved in the reproductive health of the family.

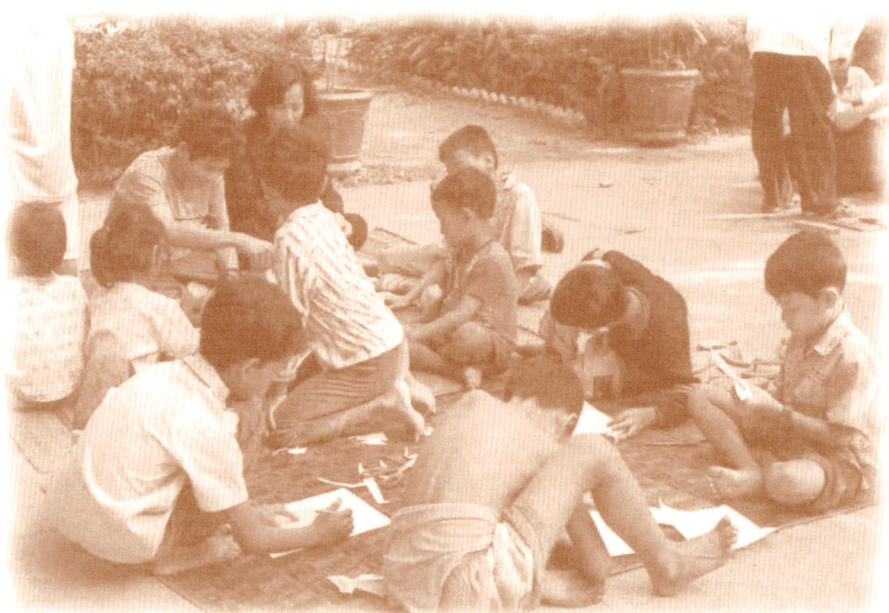

1.2 A brief history of community IMCI

September 1997 — Community IMCI was launched as a component of the IMCI strategy at the *First Global Review and Coordination Meeting on IMCI* in Santo Domingo, Dominican Republic. This meeting acknowledged the importance of families and communities in improving child health and recognized that improving the quality of care in health facilities alone would not significantly reduce childhood morbidity and mortality.

February 1998 — The Interagency Working Group on Household and Community IMCI, comprised of representatives from WHO, UNICEF, the World Bank, the United States Agency for International Development (USAID) and its implementing partners, the Department for International Development of the United Kingdom (DFID), the United Nations Foundation, and the Child Survival Collaboration and Resources (CORE) Group, was established. Its purpose is to foster a shared commitment for community IMCI; to coordinate the actions of donors, technical agencies, and implementing partners; to develop guidelines for the implementation of community IMCI; and to mobilize the necessary resources and support.

June 2000 — A consensus on the 12 key family practices and four areas of critical importance was achieved at the *International Workshop on Improving Children's Health and Nutrition in Communities,* held in Durban, South Africa. In addition, participants at the workshop agreed that the community component of IMCI is essential for any improvements to child morbidity and mortality in the next decade.

January 2001 — United States-based private voluntary organizations (PVOs), together with donors and other partners, developed a framework for household and community IMCI during the meeting on *Advancing PVO/NGO Technical Capacity and Leadership for Household and Community IMCI,* held in Baltimore, Maryland. The framework outlines three elements of community IMCI that can guide PVOs in planning, implementing, and advocating for effective community child health activities.

1.3 Development of a Western Pacific Regional Framework for Community IMCI

During the past few years, the Western Pacific Regional Office of the WHO has received a number of requests from governments for guidance on the implementation of the community component of IMCI. In order to assist governments with this component, it was determined that a clear framework would be useful that is adapted to the regional situation and that describes community IMCI and the types of activities for its implementation.

Recognizing the experience and importance of nongovernmental organizations (NGOs) in implementing community child health activities in the Region, the involvement of NGOs was sought in the early phase of the development of the Regional Framework for Community IMCI. Based on advice by the child health focal points in countries, NGOs that implement community child health activities and collaborate closely with the respective governments were identified and invited to participate in the *Regional NGO Technical Consultation on Community IMCI*[1]. During the technical consultation, NGOs discussed a variety of issues related to community IMCI and made recommendations for the regional framework.

The community IMCI framework developed by the CORE Group and Basic Support for Institutionalizing Child Survival (BASICS) II in January 2001 served as an important reference in the development of the framework for the Western Pacific Region. The two frameworks complement each other by providing insight into how to approach community IMCI from somewhat different perspectives. The CORE framework addresses the critical programming levels within a community (health facilities, private providers and volunteers, households and individuals, and non-health sectors) and seeks to maximize their use for quality preventive and curative care. Thus, the CORE framework is useful for local planning. The framework for the Western Pacific Region is composed of four areas that focus on partnerships and linkages, community participation, health information and promotion, and means for improving practices. The areas of the framework for the Western Pacific Region cut across and are essential to CORE's four programming levels, and can be used to guide the development of activities at different levels.

---

[1] Report on the "Regional NGO Technical Consultation on Community IMCI", Antipolo City, Philippines, January 29 – February 1, 2002, WHO Western Pacific Regional Office.

2. Overview of the Regional Framework for Community IMCI

Diagram 1 shows how the three components of IMCI (improved health worker skills, strengthened health system, and improved family practices) work together to improve the health status and development of the child. The components influence each other and together they have a much greater effect on the child than each one alone.

Our interest here is the third or community component of IMCI. The main focus of community IMCI is on improving key family practices, and there are four areas that contribute to improvements in these practices (partnerships and linkages; community mobilization and motivation; health information and promotion; and means for improving key family practices). The four areas are linked and mutually reinforcing. In order to have the maximum impact on key family practices, it is necessary to implement activities in all these four areas. Specific activities in each area should be designed according to the local situation and adapted to local needs.

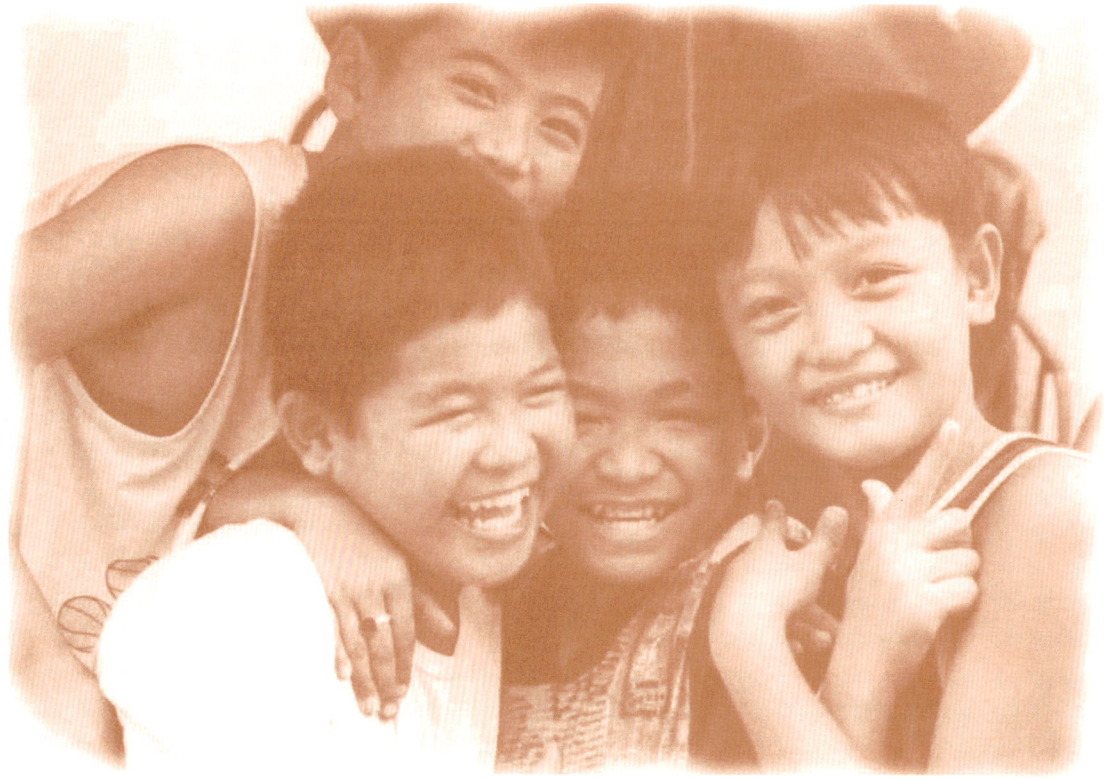

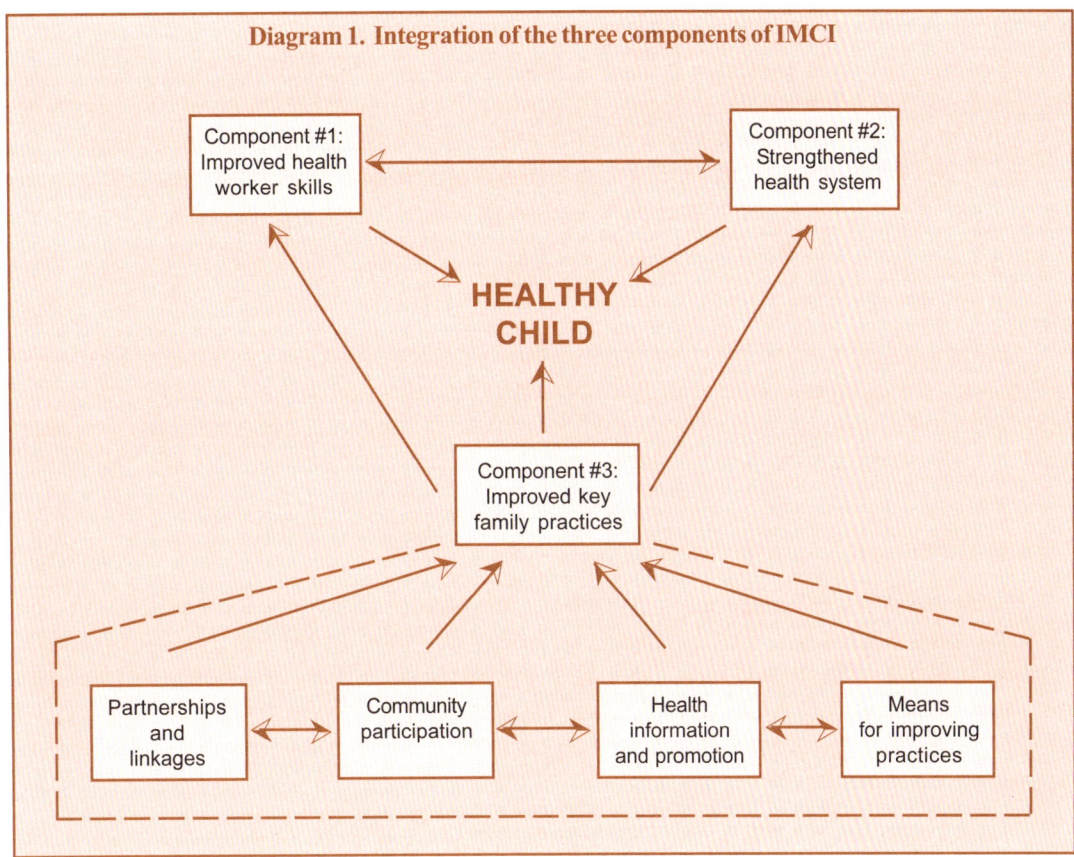

Partnerships and linkages

There are many actors involved in community IMCI planning and implementation at various levels, ranging from community members to NGO staff to Ministry of Health officials. Coordination and communication among these groups is needed to make community IMCI activities happen smoothly. This can be accomplished through the formation of partnerships.

Various types of linkages are also important to ensure a truly integrated approach at the community level. Some examples of the types of links that can be created are as follows: between different types of health programmes (e.g. IMCI and Roll Back Malaria), between different levels of the health system (e.g. centre and periphery, facilities and communities), between different government ministries (e.g. Ministry of Health and Ministry of Rural Development), and between public agencies and private companies (e.g. Ministry of Health and bednet distributors).

Community participation

Another essential factor in changing key family practices is the mobilization and motivation of community members. Communities must be involved in planning, implementing and evaluating community IMCI activities from the early stages. If communities are not asked to participate in these processes, their members are unlikely to be motivated to take part in the activities or to change their behaviours.

Health information and promotion

One important method for changing key family practices is through health information, education, communication, and promotion activities. It is advisable to use an integrated approach to behaviour change and to promote needs-based, action-oriented messages that are packaged in relevant groupings.

Means for improving practices

In some instances, community members are willing to change their behaviours but lack the means to do so. For example, they may not have access to the drugs needed to treat malaria or they may lack the funds and know-how to build a latrine for the safe disposal of faeces. In order to make the adoption of key family practices a reality, it is often necessary to devise ways for community members to gain access to the appropriate means to do so.

The four areas of community IMCI, described briefly here, are discussed in more detail in the following sections.

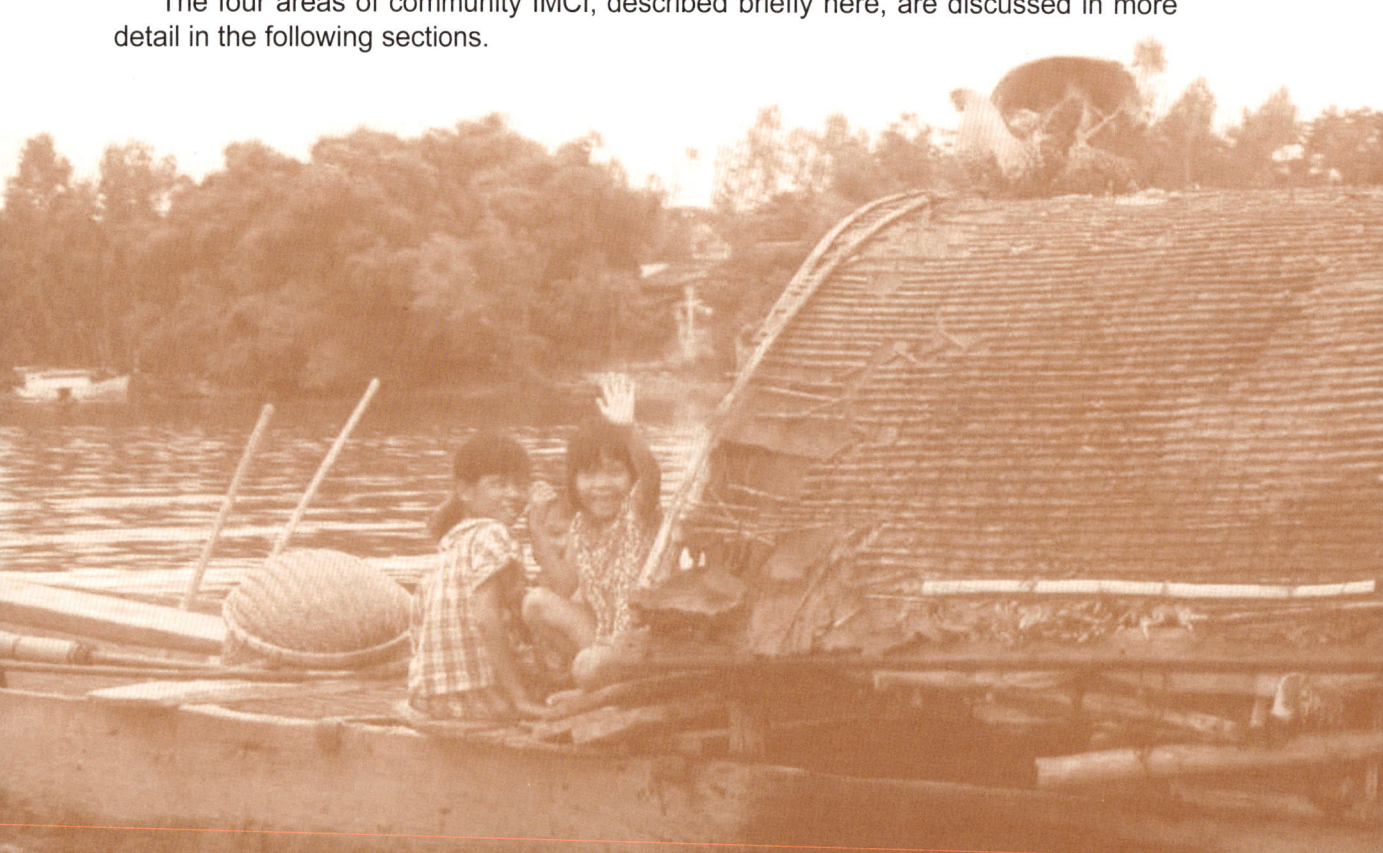

3. Description of the areas of community IMCI

3.1 Partnerships and linkages

There are a variety of types of partnerships and linkages that can contribute to improvements in the key family practices. The most important partnerships for the promotion of child health in communities are between:

- health facilities and the communities they serve;
- the government and partners (community-based organizations, local and international NGOs, bilaterals, United Nations agencies);
- different organizations implementing community activities (community-based organizations, local and international NGOs, bilaterals, United Nations agencies); and
- private and public health care providers.

The formation of partnerships and linkages is essential to community IMCI. Communities and health facilities must work together to improve the quality of health care and the use of health services. At the same time, the many local and international partners involved in the implementation of community child health activities must coordinate their efforts and develop open lines of communication among themselves and with the government. In order to achieve a multi-sectoral, integrated approach, linkages are also needed between groups working with communities on child health and those working on other health and development issues.

Partnerships and linkages of all types should be formed under the leadership of or at least with the knowledge of the Ministry of Health and its provincial and district management teams. This is necessary to ensure appropriate coordination and consistency and to make it possible for community IMCI activities to be sustained and scaled up.

3.1.1 Partnerships between health facilities and communities

In many countries, the use of public health facilities is low. Some of the reasons for low utilization are access issues (cost, distance, time), real or perceived poor quality of services, lack of knowledge about health services, and competition from the private sector. Partnerships between health facilities and communities can help to overcome some of these issues and provide benefits both to facility staff and community members.

Such linkages help health facility staff to understand the needs of communities and to adjust services to these needs. They also make facility staff more accountable to the communities they serve.

Links between health facilities and communities can take many different forms. In some countries in the Region, these links have been developed by creating Village Health Committees, Health Centre Feedback Committees, and Health Centre Co-management Committees. These committees are composed of community members and health centre staff, who meet on a periodic basis to discuss issues related to the health of the community and the functioning of the health centre. Partnerships between communities and health centres can also be facilitated by developing links between community health workers, and/or health volunteers and facilities. The information in Box 2 describes how some of these types of partnerships function and how they contribute to changes in key family practices.

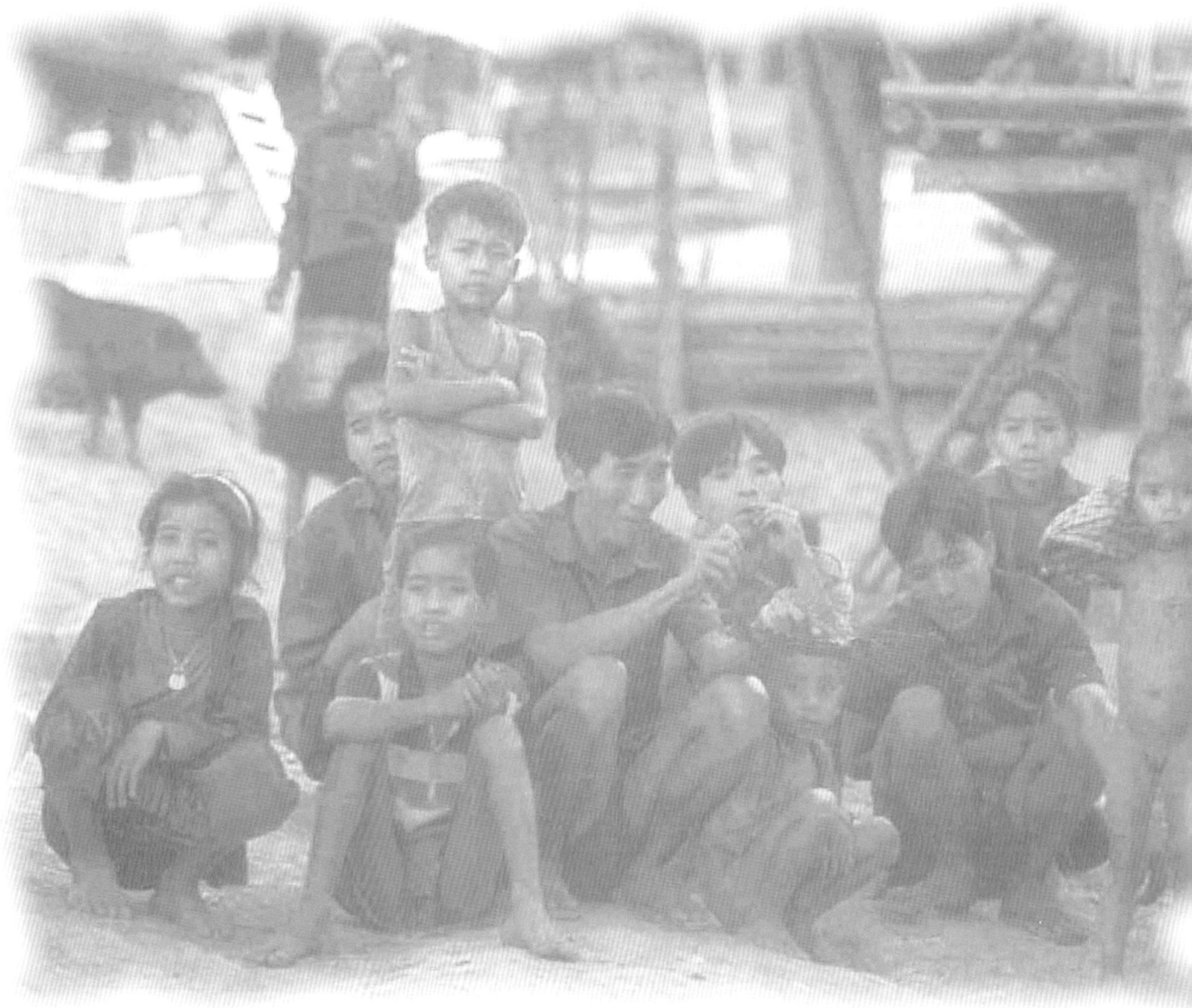

Box 2. Examples of Links between Health Facilities and Communities

Health Committees and Health Centre Feedback Committees

Health Committees and Health Centre Feedback Committees allow information to flow in both directions between health centres and communities. Community representatives on such committees meet with health centre staff to share and discuss current problems community members have with health centre services or activities. They may also help health centre staff to identify community members who are poor and should receive subsidized or free services. Health centre staff who attend committee meetings plan together with community representatives appropriate dates and times for outreach services and discuss how to improve services and other activities offered at the health centre. Community representatives then mobilize people in their villages to support and attend these services. Links between health centres and communities can also be built by asking community representatives of the Health or Feedback Committee to collect simple community-based surveillance data for analysis and use by both communities and health centre staff. By making community members more aware of the health situation of children and the types of services offered by the health centre, and by providing feedback that can improve the quality of care, Health and Feedback Committees boost the chances that parents will practice preventive behaviours and take their children to the health facility for care when they are sick.

Health Centre Co-management Committees

Co-management Committees allow community members to have input into the management and financing of health centre services. Such committees set prices for cost-recovery, manage health centre finances, and develop plans for the division of health centre income among the staff. By providing community members with direct control over the types of services offered and how they are managed, Co-management Committees give communities a sense of ownership of the health facilities that serve them. This sense of ownership makes it more likely that community members will use health facility services, thereby contributing to key family practices.

Community health workers or volunteers

Links between community health workers or volunteers and health staff are another way to strengthen partnerships between communities and health facilities. Government health staff from health centres and/or the health district can be involved in the training, support, and supervision of community health workers or volunteers. Involving health facility staff in the supervision of community health workers or volunteers ensures that they make frequent visits to communities and develop closer links with community members. Community health workers or volunteers can assist health facilities by referring community members for care and by helping health facility staff to organize and implement outreach activities. Health centre staff can provide support and feedback to these volunteers through the use of a counter-referral system, validating urgent referrals and helping volunteers check compliance with therapeutic remedies. These kinds of links provide health facility staff with a higher profile in communities. If community members trust the volunteer and know the staff of health facilities, they may be more likely to use their services. Such links are also helpful to health facilities because referrals by community health workers or volunteers increase the number of patients, and the help of community health workers or volunteers makes outreach sessions go more smoothly.

3.1.2 Partnerships between government and partners

In every country, there are many agencies already involved in community child health activities. The main actors include government institutions, community-based organizations, local and international NGOs, bilateral organizations, and United Nations agencies. It is advisable for the government to coordinate the activities of all actors by developing partnerships with implementing agencies. Partnerships between the government and interested agencies can be organized through, for example, a Community IMCI Sub-group of the IMCI Working Group at the national level and through Community IMCI Coordination Committees at provincial and/or district level. Participation in these types of groups or committees allows the government and partners to have joint input into the implementation process and to stay informed about activities carried out by each party. The composition and function of these groups are described in Box 3.

Box 3. Mechanisms for coordinating partnerships between government and partners

Community IMCI Sub-group

At the national level, the Community IMCI Sub-group should include representatives from all government ministries and institutions that have child health activities at community level and from all partners involved in decision-making about or implementation of community child health activities. The main purpose of the sub-group is to assist with the development of a strategy for community IMCI at the national level, including budgeting and identifying sources of funds, and to coordinate planned activities. This group can work to ensure a certain level of nationwide standardization of messages, activities, and indicators related to child health. It can also develop standards about who should be involved in community child health activities (e.g. community health workers, health volunteers, traditional birth attendants, traditional healers, private providers, etc.) and the roles of each of these providers.

Provincial and/or District Community IMCI Coordination Committee

At the provincial or district level, provincial or district health authorities, health facility staff, and local partners (e.g. community-based organizations, local and international NGOs, UNICEF, etc.) may choose to form a committee for the planning and coordination of community IMCI activities. This committee should include representatives from the community and other important groups, such as private providers or traditional healers. The purpose of this committee is to coordinate community IMCI activities at the provincial or district level. Some of the activities that a provincial or district level committee might carry out are detailed in Annex 1. This type of committee ensures that local government staff, partners, and community members work together to plan and carry out child health activities that fit the local situation and that can be sustained.

3.1.3 Partnerships between different groups and organizations implementing community activities

Partnerships between different organizations or agencies implementing community activities may take a variety of forms and serve different purposes. Some examples of such partnerships are as follows:

- Community-based organizations and local and international NGOs within one country can form a community IMCI network that shares information about and experiences with community IMCI activities. Group members can help each other solve problems related to implementation, share tools (e.g., training materials or data collection forms) and/or develop collaborative activities. These organizations can also form partnerships between themselves for actual implementation of community IMCI activities. Such partnerships can exist between organizations working in different geographical areas in the same province or district or between organizations with complementary programmes in the same geographical area.

- In some countries, an umbrella organization for agencies implementing health activities already exists. In these cases, agencies or organizations involved in community child health activities can form a Community IMCI Committee or Working Group within the umbrella organization.

- Bilateral agencies can create partnerships at a variety of levels in order to fund community IMCI activities. They may partner with and provide funding to NGOs, governments, and regional groups of countries.

- United Nations agencies can develop partnerships between themselves to provide technical assistance to the government or with local and international NGOs to develop joint plans for implementation.

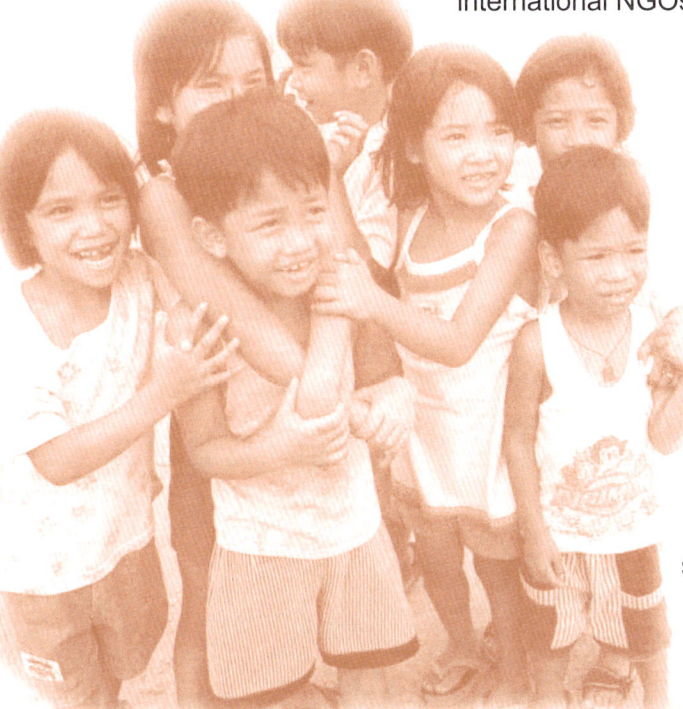

Partnerships between organizations implementing community activities contribute to the improvement of key family practices by providing a forum for problem-solving related to implementation, by preventing overlapping or conflicting activities in communities, and by directing the flow of funding for community child health activities. These types of partnerships also facilitate the implementation of a coordinated national community IMCI strategy that involves multiple partners and a variety of approaches to improve selected practices.

3.1.4 Partnerships between private and public health care providers

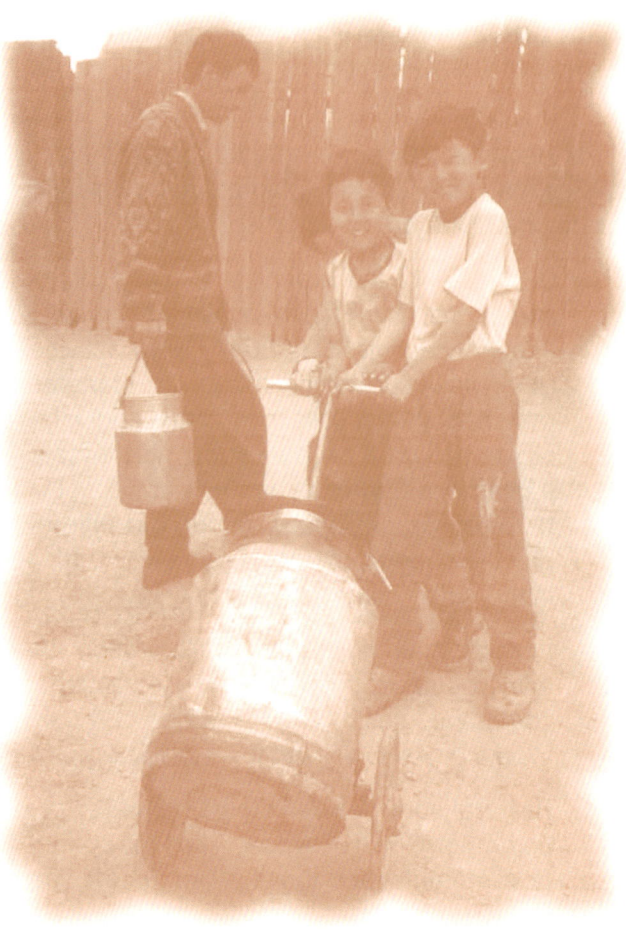

Forming partnerships between private and public health care providers is a sensitive topic in some countries. However, the reality is that private providers exist in most communities and their services and advice are sought regularly. One way to link private and public health care providers is to train private providers to refer serious cases to public health facilities and to counsel clients on prevention and home care for childhood illnesses. Links between these two groups could also be made by holding meetings to exchange experiences on working with communities, through sharing of health education and training materials or by hosting health days on needs-based topics. In some countries, it may be possible for private and public health care providers to conduct joint community IMCI activities or for private providers to sponsor some activities led by the public sector.

3.1.5 Collaboration within the Ministry of Health and between government ministries

In addition to the types of partnerships outlined above, there are some important linkages that may need to be formed or reinforced in order to create a multi-sectoral and integrated approach to community IMCI. The most important linkages for IMCI are between different programmes within the Ministry of Health. All of the programmes that formerly provided (or continue to provide) services to children in a vertical manner need to be involved in a process of developing an integrated package of messages and community-based activities for child health. The section(s) of the Ministry of Health responsible for community activities, outreach and health education or promotion should be included in these efforts.

3.3 Health information and promotion

Health information and promotion can have a direct impact on improving key family practices by providing community members with new health knowledge, sharing examples of preventive behaviours and appropriate caring practices, and enabling caretakers to practise these new behaviours. Using health communication to change behaviour is not a new idea or approach. The key issues for health communication related to community IMCI are the integration of health messages that were previously provided by many partners and vertical programmes, and the development of a "standard" package of messages.

To develop a standard set of messages related to the 12 key family practices, a review of existing qualitative and quantitative research on child health knowledge, attitudes, and practices should be undertaken. If necessary, additional research can be conducted to fill in any gaps in the available data. Based on the information obtained or collected, an integrated behaviour change strategy for child health should be developed at the appropriate level. Some ideas for the integration of messages and behaviours are the use of guided counselling materials, seasonal promotion of behaviours, and grouping related behaviours together (see Box 5).

It is important that messages coming from different channels and different partners are the same. To ensure this, the behaviour change strategy should be developed and/or reviewed by the Community IMCI Sub-group, and agreed upon by its members and other key partners.

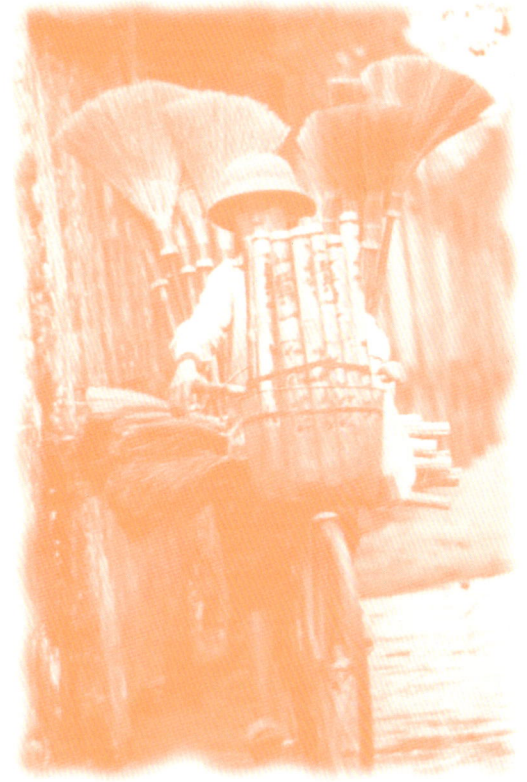

Messages should be targeted at specific actions community members can or should take rather than providing general health knowledge. It is not advisable to introduce messages on all of the key family practices at one time. In fact, the sub-group should select a few practices to focus on at first and make a plan to phase in behaviour change communication on the other practices over time. It may be necessary to adapt materials developed nationally to fit with different practices or customs in some districts; however the messages provided should remain the same.

A variety of channels for health communication should be used. This ensures that community members hear the same messages multiple times from different sources. In addition to face-to-face communication provided through facility- and community-based individuals, messages can be spread through mass media (radio, television, printed materials), popular methods (dramas, songs, puppet shows, group discussions), and participatory approaches. Introducing health promotion messages using participatory methods allows community members to make the links between their own practices and their children's health, and helps them to develop a commitment to change.

Face-to-face health communication can be provided to community members through public health workers, community health workers or volunteers, traditional birth attendants, traditional healers, drug sellers, other private providers, religious leaders, etc. Training for public health workers and community members who provide health information is necessary. They may require training both on the health information itself and on counselling skills. Both health workers and community volunteers need regular supervision, support and feedback on their health promotion and counselling skills, and health workers should be encouraged to recognize health promotion as a key element of their clinical practice.

During face-to-face communication sessions in communities, it is helpful to provide opportunities for community members to see or practice new behaviours. This can be done through the modelling of appropriate practices by community-based individuals, through activities such as cooking demonstrations and oral rehydration salts (ORS) mixing sessions, and through peer-led sessions where actual practice with counselling can occur.

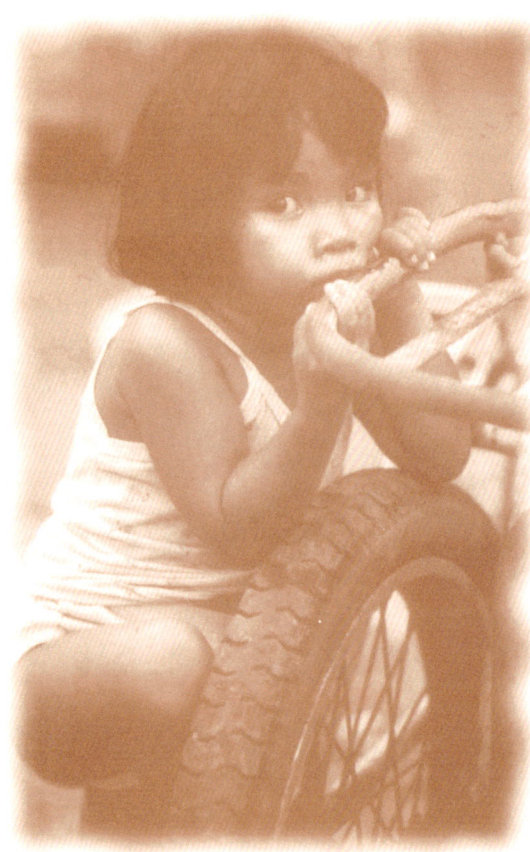

In some countries, it may be necessary to focus a portion of the health communication efforts on changing harmful practices, for example, those related to the inappropriate use of drugs. When drugs are available in communities, they may be provided to children in a harmful manner. Both community members and drug sellers or other private providers should be educated about the dangerous nature of these practices.

In areas of a country that have limited access to health facilities, governments or NGOs may train community health workers to make simple assessments of childhood illnesses and refer cases that cannot be managed locally to higher level health facilities. Community health workers can also provide counselling on basic preventive and promotive practices for illnesses that can be locally managed and can provide information about services available at health centres.

> **Box 5. Integrated behaviour change strategies**
>
> In developing a strategy for promoting the key family practices, it is important to think about who will perform the promoted behaviours, when the behaviours will be performed, and where they will take place. With this information in mind, it is possible to determine which messages should be introduced, when, in what combinations, and through which channels. It is essential to present messages in small action-oriented doses so the behaviours can be absorbed and tried out before new messages are added. A few examples of ways to provide integrated messages in "bite-size" pieces are as follows:
>
> *Guided counselling materials*
>
> Guided counselling materials are often packaged as a flipchart or set of counselling cards. The person who uses the cards (community health worker, volunteer, private provider, health worker) is trained to find out from the mother or caretaker which issue(s) are relevant each time they meet. The "counsellor" then uses the appropriate pages of the counselling materials to tailor the session to the mother's needs. For example, if the child has diarrhoea, the counsellor may talk to the mother about feeding and fluids during diarrhoea, signs that indicate the child should be taken to a health facility, and actions for preventing diarrhoea in the future.
>
> *Seasonal promotion of behaviours*
>
> Many diseases or health problems occur more frequently during certain times of the year. A practical way to link messages to action is to introduce relevant messages at the beginning of the season when a disease or type of illness becomes more prevalent. For example, in areas where there is a dengue fever risk, community health workers can promote the importance of covering containers that hold standing water and clearing garbage from around the house at the beginning of the rainy season. Promoting behaviours by season also helps to determine when different messages should be introduced, and an annual calendar can be developed.
>
> *Grouping related behaviours*
>
> It may be helpful to group related behaviours together and to promote them as a package. For example, community health workers could promote the behaviours related to care of illness and care-seeking (e.g. recognition of illness, home care, care-seeking outside the home, and following instructions of the health worker) as one group of important behaviours.

3.4 Means for improving key practices

In many communities, families do not have access to services or commodities that they need to be able to undertake some of the key family practices. For example, a family that lives in a malaria-endemic area where no insecticide-treated bednets are available or where they are too expensive for the family to afford cannot adopt the practice of protecting their children from malaria by using bednets. In such cases, it may be necessary to improve access to and availability of the means for improving practices. Table 1 outlines some of the means for improving practices that may be difficult to access and gives examples of how access could be increased.

Table 1. Improving practices

Means for improving practices	Possible ways to increase access and availability
Commodities: e.g. insecticide-treated bednets, essential medicines	• Invite private companies to distribute and sell the necessary commodities • Support community groups to develop businesses for retreating bednets with insecticide • Develop a social marketing system for selling commodities through private vendors • Sell commodities through community health workers, volunteers, traditional birth attendants or others • Sell or provide commodities through health workers during outreach visits to communities • Develop a drug revolving fund for private vendors, community-based volunteers, or health workers to obtain additional quantities of drugs and other supplies • Set up community drug boxes or community pharmacies
Infrastructure: e.g. water supply and sanitation, transportation	• Provide community members with blueprints and materials to build low-cost latrines • Subsidize the cost of latrines through a revolving fund • Promote low-cost, appropriate technology solutions to water supply and sanitation needs • Invite other agencies or partners to implement water and sanitation activities • Develop community-based plans to provide emergency transportation to health facilities • Create a community revolving fund to pay for emergency transportation
Services at health facilities: e.g. curative care, preventive care (micronutrients, immunization)	• Introduce an exemption scheme whereby community members who are unable to pay receive health services at subsidized rates or for free • Allow community members to be involved in setting fees for health services (e.g. through management committees)

<td colspan="2" align="center">**Table 1. Improving practices (continued...)**</td>
Means for improving practices	**Possible ways to increase access and availability**
	• Support community committees to define health facility quality standards that will increase use of facility services • Develop a system (possibly using slips) for community health workers, volunteers, traditional birth attendants, drug sellers, etc. involved in community child health activities to refer children to health facilities
Services in the community: e.g. distribution of vitamin A, growth monitoring	• Provide micronutrient supplementation and immunization services through outreach in hard-to-reach communities • In countries where the government policy allows it, train and equip community health workers, traditional birth attendants, and/or private providers to assess and treat illnesses (such as acute respiratory infections in areas where access to health facilities is very difficult • Train and equip community health workers, traditional birth attendants, and/or private providers to distribute Vitamin A to children and post-partum mothers, iron/folate tablets to pregnant women, iodized salt, ORS packets, condoms, etc. • Train community health workers, traditional birth attendants, and/or private providers to conduct growth monitoring and promotion activities
Health information and education: e.g. counselling and health education services	• Distribute information, education and communication (IEC) materials to community health workers, volunteers, traditional birth attendants, private providers, etc. so they can provide health education and counselling services on preventive and caring practices to community members • Develop a system for replacing community health workers or volunteers who decide to discontinue their activities • Provide incentives and continuing education to community health workers or volunteers to prevent them from dropping out • Seek out free radio time and newspaper space for disseminating critical maternal and child health messages • Invite local drama and choral groups to perform health messages at outreach services, health days, and maternal and child health clinic times at health facilities • Set up community scoreboards to display community-based data on the health situation of women and children.

4. Links within the framework and between the three IMCI components

4.1 Links between the areas of the framework

The four areas of the framework outlined above are closely linked and mutually reinforcing. The relationship between the four areas is more complex than can be shown on the framework diagram. In essence, each area is linked to all the other areas. The following paragraphs give just a few examples of how the different areas are interrelated.

Community participation can serve as a means of facilitating activities related to the other three areas. Community mobilization and motivation is needed for partnerships between health facilities and communities to function, especially in places where community members are asked to provide feedback on or manage health facility services. Community participation is also required to increase access to the means for improving practices. For example, community input is necessary in the development of a community-based plan for transportation to health facilities. Community mobilization and motivation is essential for health education and promotion to be successful. Community members are often recruited and trained to counsel their neighbours on important child health issues. The motivation of community members is needed both for them to attend health education sessions conducted by community health workers and to take action to try or to adopt new behaviours.

Health information and promotion is linked to increasing access to the means for improving practices. Through health education, community members can be informed about the types of services available at health facilities or about the importance of obtaining commodities that can protect children from health problems.

Partnerships play an important role in influencing the type of health information and promotion that is received by community members. Through a national level Community IMCI Sub-group, messages can be standardized and plans for use of different communication channels determined. Partnerships may also be needed to increase access to means for improving practices. For example, partnerships between the Ministry of Health and other ministries or between different implementing organizations may make it possible to provide infrastructure (e.g. latrines) in communities that need it.

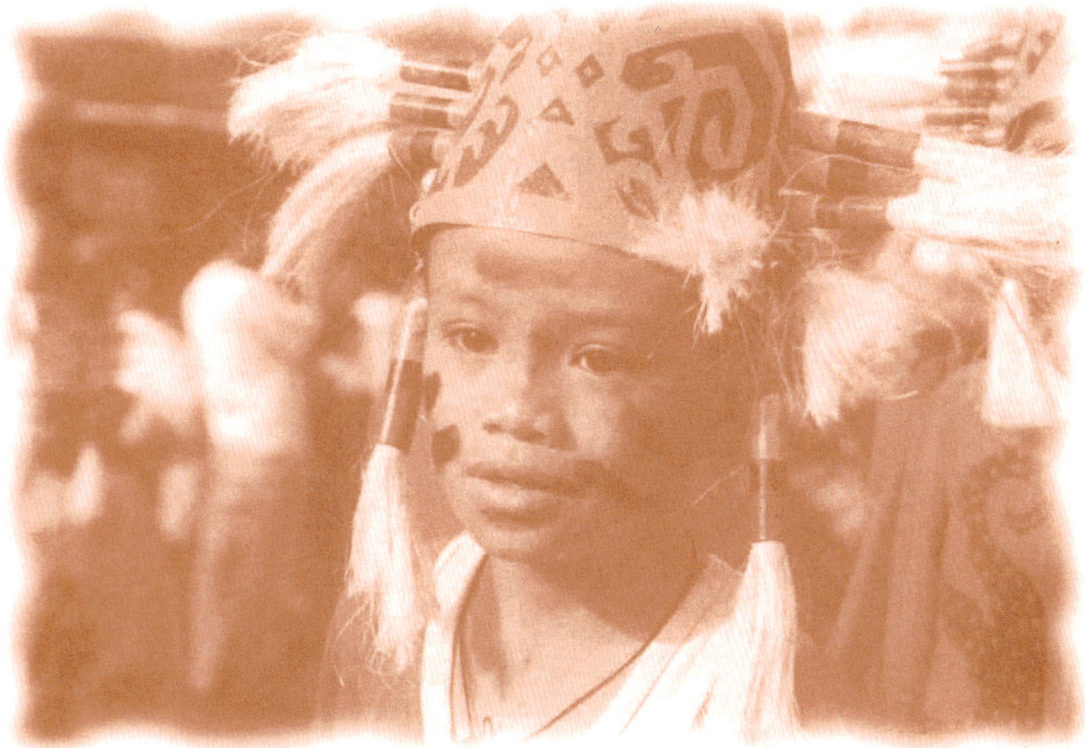

4.2 Links between the three components of the IMCI strategy

The three components of IMCI are linked, and they support each other when fully implemented (see Diagram 2). When Components 1 (Improved health worker skills) and 2 (Strengthened health system) are in place, they can help to reinforce some aspects of Component 3 (Improved key family practices). For example, trained health workers can contribute to health information and promotion in the community by providing counselling to mothers during visits to the health facility or during outreach sessions. Strengthening the quality of services at health facilities makes those services more desirable and makes it easier to mobilize community members to use them.

Parts of IMCI Component 3 also contribute to the other two components. Partnerships between health facilities and communities help to strengthen the health system and improve the quality of services. Community mobilization and health education at the community level make it easier for health workers to conduct outreach activities and also make community members more likely to use health services.

Because of the synergy between the components of IMCI, it is important for governments to plan to have all three components in place within a reasonable period of time. When all three components are functioning simultaneously, they strengthen each other and may have a greater impact on child morbidity and mortality.

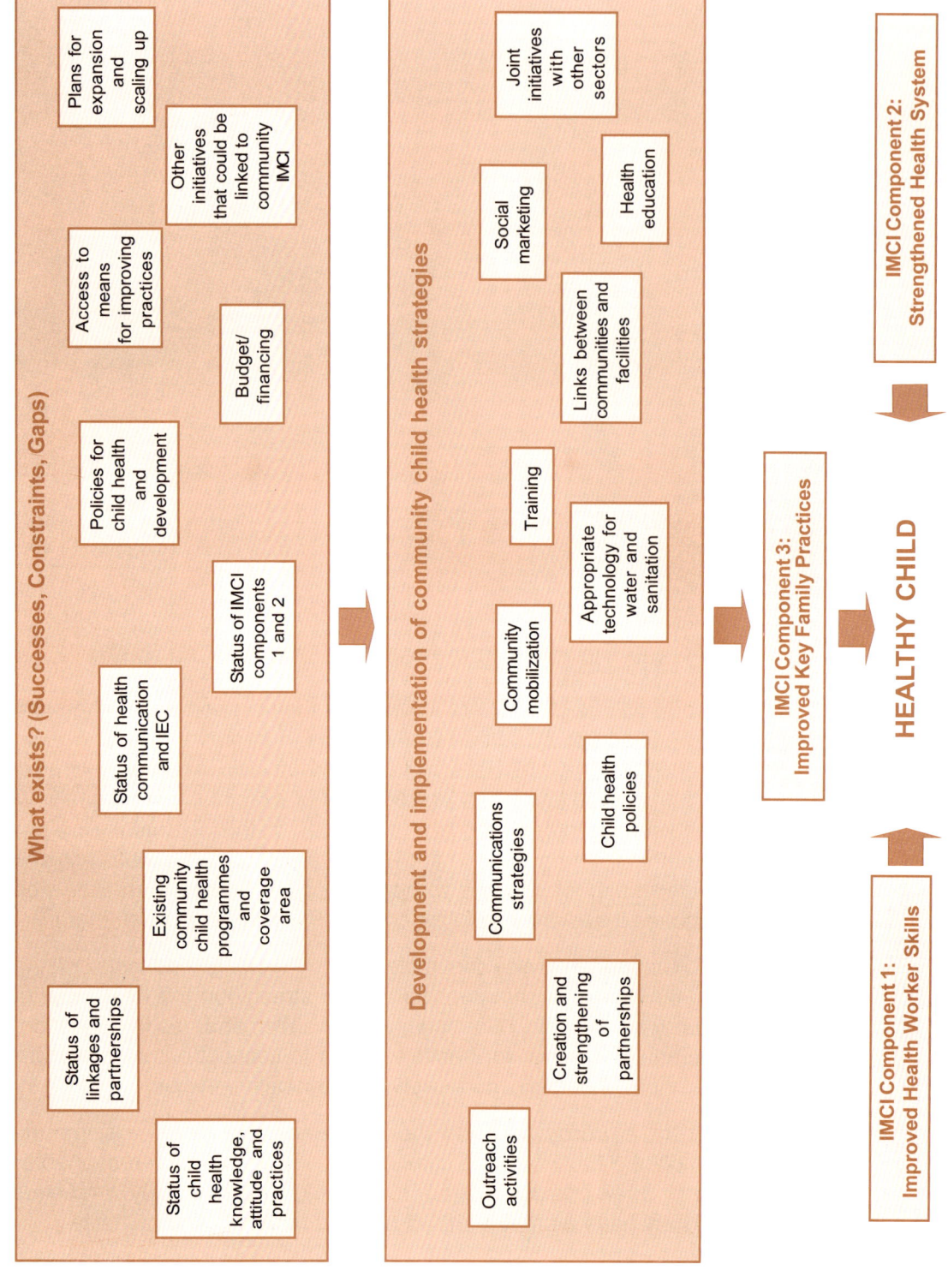

Diagram 2. Planning, development and implementation of community IMCI

5. Roles of different actors in community IMCI implementation

There are many types of people or actors involved in the implementation of community IMCI activities. The types of actors vary from country to country and their roles may differ depending on the local structures. The table below provides some general ideas and guidelines about the roles of each group.

Table 2. Roles and responsibilities of each implementing actor

Type of implementing actor	Roles and responsibilities
Government at national level (e.g. Ministry of Health, Child Health Institute, and other national institutions)	• Take overall responsibility for community IMCI coordination and policy development • Guide the national planning process for community IMCI • Communicate national decisions regarding community IMCI to the provincial and district levels • Provide assistance to provincial and district levels for planning and implementation • Facilitate the formation of a Community IMCI Sub-group, including representatives from all partners, relevant departments of the Ministry of Health, and other government institutions • Coordinate the geographical areas of implementation among partners • Ensure that health messages are standardized • Ensure that laws and regulations as well as their enforcement support community IMCI interventions • Identify support for community IMCI activities in geographical areas without support • Guide the evaluation process
Government at provincial and/or district level	• Facilitate the formation of a provincial and/or district Community IMCI Coordination Committee • Guide the provincial, district and community planning process, including the development of written plans at each level

Type of implementing actor	Roles and responsibilities
	• Take responsibility for coordinating community IMCI implementation, including administrative and financial management • Ensure that all three components of IMCI are implemented and mutually reinforcing • Work with partners to mobilize communities through participatory methods/activities • Adapt/develop baseline indicators, monitor programme activities and periodically evaluate progress
Government at local level	• Act as liaison between district and communities • Support communities in the implementation of activities • Make decisions about funding for health activities, including stipends for community health workers (in some countries)
Health workers	• Train, support and supervise community health workers or volunteers who provide health information in communities • Coordinate the activities of community health workers or volunteers • Provide outreach services in communities (immunization, vitamin A) • Counsel mothers about treatment, home care, and prevention during visits to health facilities and during outreach visits • Collaborate with Health Committees, Feedback Committees and/or Co-management Committees to improve the quality and functioning of health services • Collect, analyse and use health data to make changes in programme strategies or activities
Community health workers or community-based volunteers	• Provide health education and conduct health promotion activities that promote key family practices and proper home care • Refer community members to health services as necessary • Assist with community mobilization activities

Table 2. Roles and responsibilities of each implementing actor (continued...)

Table 2. Roles and responsibilities of each implementing actor (continued...)	
Type of implementing actor	**Roles and responsibilities**
	• Sell or provide health commodities (in some countries) • Collect simple health data and report it back to communities and to health facilities • Provide feedback to health facilities to improve their quality and use by community members
Private providers (e.g. traditional birth attendants, drug sellers, traditional healers, pharmacists, etc.)	• Promote the key family practices and preventive actions • Counsel clients on home care for illnesses • Refer community members to health services as necessary • Reduce harmful use of drugs
Village leaders, Village Development Committees	• Mobilize community participation in child health activities • Participate in community IMCI strategy development and planning
Health Committees (e.g. Health Centre Feedback Committee, Health Centre Co-management Committee, Village Health Committee)	• Provide feedback to health centres about problems community members have with services • Ensure that community members know what types of services are available at health facilities and when outreach activities will take place • Serve as conduit of information between health facilities and communities • Assist in decision-making about the functioning and management of health services • Work towards the improvement of the quality of services
Local and international NGOs	• Participate in Community IMCI Sub-groups or Coordinating Committees at all levels • Collaborate with the members of the Community IMCI Sub-group to standardize health messages • Participate in national and provincial/district planning processes, including identification of priorities • Serve as implementing partners of community IMCI activities

Table 2. Roles and responsibilities of each implementing actor (continued...)	
Type of implementing actor	**Roles and responsibilities**
	• Provide financial and technical support for community IMCI activities
	• Foster links or develop strategies to link communities and health facilities
	• Build government capacity (at all levels) to implement and coordinate community IMCI activities
	• Advocate to government regarding policies and implementation strategies
	• Test new or innovative approaches to improving key family practices
United Nations agencies (e.g. WHO and UNICEF)	• Facilitate formation of partnerships/communication between government and implementing partners
	• Provide technical support and advice to governments on IMCI implementation
	• Share information about community IMCI activities
	• Act as an implementing agency for community IMCI activities (UNICEF)
	• Participate in national and provincial/district planning processes, including identification of priorities
	• Build government capacity (at all levels) to implement and coordinate community IMCI activities
	• Assist in the organization of national and local networks of NGOs to coordinate their involvement in community IMCI
Bilaterals	• Coordinate support for community IMCI based on government priorities
	• Facilitate formation of partnerships/communication between government and implementing partners
	• Build government capacity (at all levels) to implement and coordinate community approaches
	• Assist in the organization of national and local networks of NGOs to coordinate their involvement in community IMCI.

6. Guiding principles for community IMCI planning and implementation

This section describes the principles that guide community IMCI planning and implementation. These principles should be considered carefully and referred to regularly during the process of developing a national strategy for community IMCI, while planning at the provincial and/or district level, and during the implementation of community-based activities.

- **Consultation between partners at all levels is required for successful planning, implementation and coordination of community activities.**

    Because so many players are involved in decision-making or provision of services at the community level, partnerships and open communication are prerequisites for the implementation of community child health activities. The Ministry of Health and its structures at different levels should play a leading role in the formation of partnerships. All types of partners, governmental, nongovernmental, bilateral, and multilateral, should be involved in consultations about community IMCI at the national level. At the district and local levels, appropriate partners, including community members, should be included in planning, implementing, and evaluating community child health activities. In preparing for meetings of partners at all levels, efforts should be made to ensure that participants are decision-makers or are able to report quickly to decision-makers. This improves communication and prevents meetings where no decisions are made.

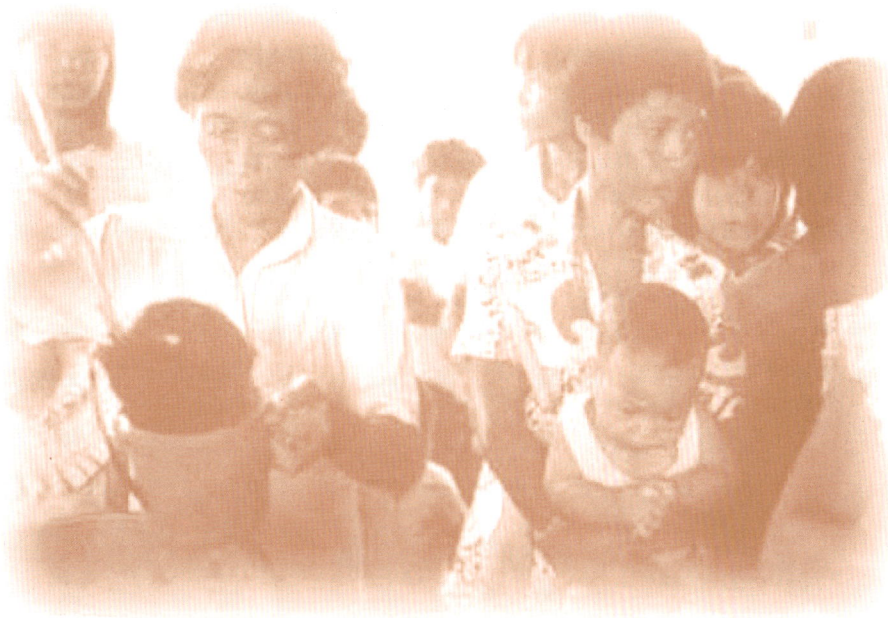

- **Participatory processes should be used at various levels, to involve communities and promote community ownership.**

    Participatory approaches can be used to promote ownership of community IMCI activities among partners at the national and district levels. However, it is even more important to involve community members in assessment and planning from an early stage through participatory methods. By including communities in the process, their level of ownership for community IMCI activities is increased.

- **Community IMCI should build upon activities that are already taking place in communities.**

    It is clear that a variety of community child health activities are already taking place in many countries in the Region. These may be supported by governments, NGOs, United Nations agencies, bilateral agencies and other implementing partners or they may simply be community-owned. In planning for community IMCI implementation, existing activities should be reviewed and incorporated or expanded within community IMCI. There is no need to start with a clean slate when activities are already taking place in communities or districts. In fact, an effort should be made to avoid developing and implementing new cadres of human resources (e.g. community health workers where none already exist) or other structures that may be effective in the short term, but are expensive and difficult to manage in the long run.

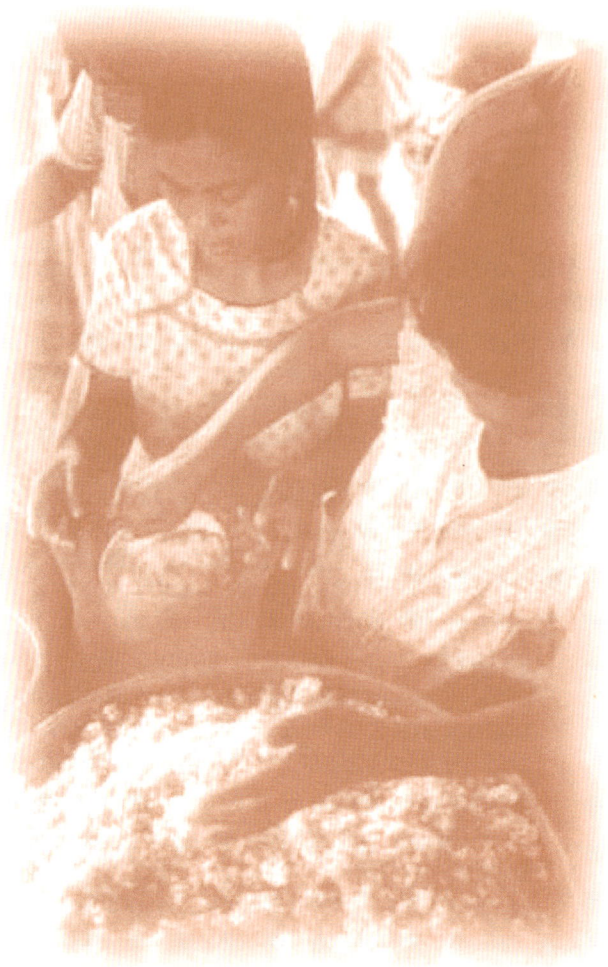

- **There are multiple entry points for initiating community IMCI activities.**

It is possible to approach community IMCI implementation from a variety of different entry points. This could mean that different parts of community IMCI (as outlined in this framework) or different groups of key family practices are phased in over time. Multiple entry points could also mean that community IMCI activities start from a non-health intervention. For example, a government ministry or an NGO project may enter a community and develop a relationship with that community through an income-generating or credit activity. Once established, the community structures created for the credit activity could be used to promote key family practices. In some areas, this type of "back door" approach may be even more effective than a purely health intervention.

- **It is necessary to implement activities in all the four areas of community IMCI outlined in this framework.**

The four areas of community IMCI outlined in this framework are closely linked and mutually reinforcing. Although the actual way each area is implemented may be different from country to country and even in different geographic areas within one country, all four areas are needed to fully promote and improve the key family practices.

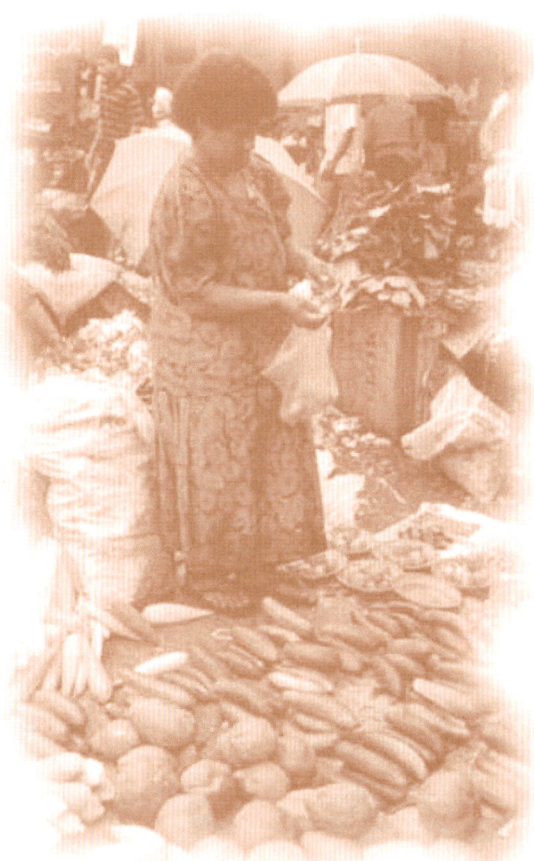

- **The four areas of community IMCI outlined in the framework can be introduced in a phased manner.**

It may not be possible to introduce activities in all four areas of community IMCI simultaneously. In fact, it may be helpful to start with the development of partnerships and community mobilization, and later add the other two areas. Access to the means for improving practices may be the most complicated area to address, and in some places may require formulating policies prior to implementation.

- **The promotion of key family practices can be introduced in a phased manner.**

Each of the 12 key family and community practices is composed of several steps. In order to avoid information overload at the community level, it is strongly recommended to phase in the introduction of key family practices. It is advisable to select a few practices to start with based on the most urgent needs, to phase in groups of related practices, or to start with practices that are easiest for parents to change.

- **Clear government policies related to community IMCI issues are needed to facilitate implementation.**

    It is helpful and may be necessary to have clear government policies related to community IMCI. For example, in some countries, there are laws acknowledging the role of community health workers in primary health care and giving them the right to provide simple health services in remote areas. These kinds of laws make the community health workers' role clear and simplify the introduction of community IMCI activities that involve them. Other types of policies might be needed on issues such as the sale of drugs by untrained providers, the role of private providers or community-based providers in the treatment of childhood illnesses, or the provision of Vitamin A capsules. It is easier to standardize implementation of community IMCI once such policies are in place.

As indicated in the first step, representatives from the community should be asked to participate in planning at the provincial or district (and possibly at the national) level. This means that community representatives should be involved in all of the steps of provincial or district planning outlined above, including the situation analysis. At the community level, collection and analysis of data can be done using a variety of methods, including those such as PLA (see page 18). Use of participatory methods provides an excellent opportunity for combining strategy development and planning with community mobilization. Once data are collected, community members should also be involved in the selection of interventions and the development of a local plan of action.

A table with more details about the activities related to each of the steps for national, provincial or district, and community planning for community IMCI is included in Annex 1. This table is a modified version of a planning table developed by the global Interagency Working Group on Household and Community IMCI.

The order of planning by level can be determined in each country. Some countries may choose to plan at the national level before starting provincial or district and community planning. However, it is also possible to do national, provincial or district, and community planning simultaneously. In some countries, it may be necessary to develop capacity at an intermediate level to allow regions or provinces to function autonomously. It is recommended that district and community level planning be conducted concurrently.

It is important to remember that planning at all levels is necessary. However, as actions to improve child health take place in the community and district, attention should be paid to the development of plans at these levels and efforts made to ensure that local plans are appropriate and feasible.

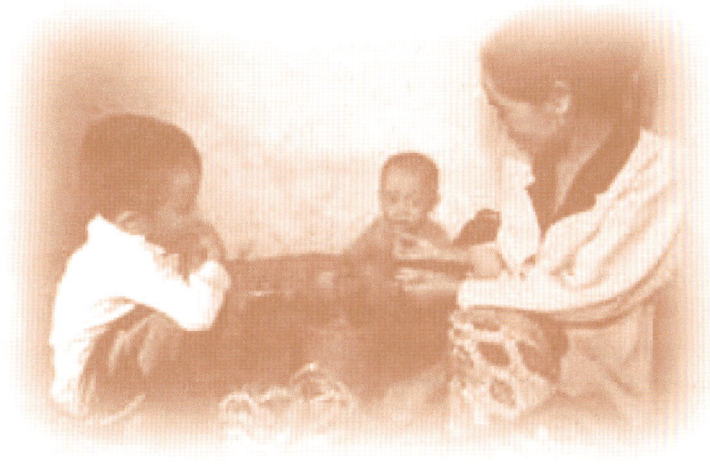

8. Sustainability and scaling-up

8.1 Sustainability

The issue of sustaining community child health activities should be considered from the beginning of the planning and strategy development process. Sustainability should be discussed by community IMCI coordination groups at all levels, and should be addressed in the national, provincial and district level strategies. Inclusion of community IMCI activities in national, provincial and district budgets shows the government's willingness to reduce dependence on outside financing and makes the community IMCI strategy more sustainable.

Some specific ways to increase the sustainability of community IMCI activities are to:

- build capacity of district and health facility staff to plan and implement community child health activities;
- build capacity of community-based structures (e.g. village health committee, village development committee, etc.) to take over activities;
- build community ownership of and demand for activities;
- build ownership of community IMCI activities among partners at all levels;
- build capacity of a local NGO or other community-based organizations to manage and sustain community activities;
- link community child health activities to other established community-based efforts (e.g. micro-credit, agriculture);
- develop policies that institutionalize and support community-based activities at all levels; and
- allocate resources on an annual basis for community activities.

Building capacity at the local level is important to ensure that community-based activities continue. However, capacity alone cannot sustain activities. It must be supported by a demand for the activities and by some type of financing (e.g. direct budget allocation or links to micro-credit/ income-generating activities). Sustainability of community IMCI activities can also be greatly facilitated by appropriate policies. For example, a policy that outlines the role of community health workers and describes a means for their support can have an important influence on the sustainability of the activities carried out.

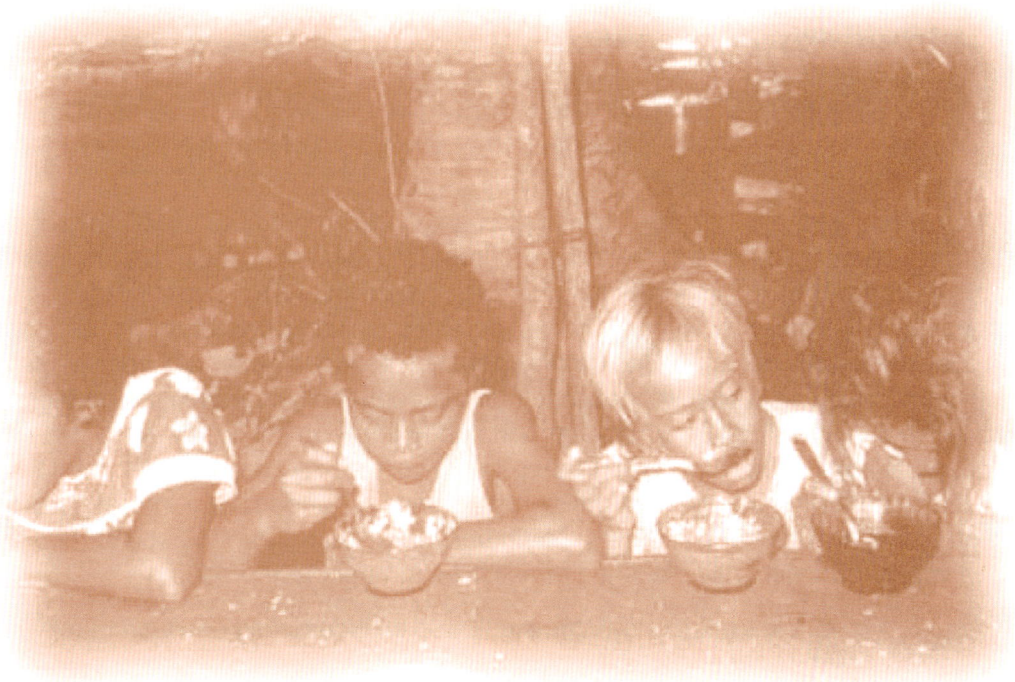

8.2 Scaling up

Scaling up community IMCI activities is essential if they are to have a significant impact on infant and child mortality. Community IMCI can be scaled up by adding activities related to more of the key family practices to existing programmes and by expanding activities to cover new geographical areas. In general, community IMCI should be implemented in the same geographic areas as the other two components of the IMCI strategy, and expansion of all three components should take place simultaneously, if possible.

Community IMCI coordination groups should plan for scaling up community activities early in the planning process, and these should be outlined in strategies at all levels. Once the pilot experiences with community IMCI implementation have been reviewed, and successes and constraints discussed with partners, a plan can be made for linking successful community IMCI activities that are supported by different partners, and expanding them to cover more areas of the country where the IMCI strategy is implemented. The partners, including community representatives, should be involved in the process and agree on the types of community IMCI activities that would be included in a more or less "standard package" for scaling up. One way to spread successful approaches or experiences is to have strong implementing partners mentor government staff or staff of other agencies in new geographical areas. It is also necessary to allocate or identify funding for expansion. This may require advocacy with donors to make IMCI, in general, and community IMCI, specifically, a priority.

9. Monitoring and evaluation

Monitoring and evaluation of the implementation of community IMCI activities is important in order to be able to measure progress and to identify and solve any possible problems as they occur. Within the national strategy, it is useful to have a list of indicators for measuring the impact of community IMCI activities, including indicators of sustainability and the process of scaling up. Indicators should be selected based on what is relevant in a given country. It is also important to make sure that all implementing partners are involved in the selection of indicators and that they agree to collect the necessary data to measure them. This may mean that on-going community programmes need to add new indicators or modify some of their existing ones. Standardizing indicators across implementing agencies will allow the Community IMCI Sub-group to get a clear picture of the impact of community child health activities throughout the country.

At global level, the Interagency Working Group on Household and Community IMCI has identified and agreed upon a list of priority indicators and proposed supplemental measures for IMCI at the household level. The indicators are designed to measure progress in behavioural change toward the key family practices and in programme implementation. The lists of indicators can be found in Annex 2.

In addition to considering indicators for monitoring and evaluation, the Ministry of Health and its partners involved in community IMCI implementation may want to develop some plans for operations research. Community IMCI is a new field in many countries, so it may be worthwhile to conduct research to measure the impact of specific activities. Data gained from operations research can be used to identify important lessons from field experience and may contribute to sustainability and assist in plans for scaling up.

Annex 1

Table of planning process

Child health in communities: A guide for developing implementation strategies

A. National level planning process for community IMCI

Step/Phase	Activities	Outcomes	Comments
1. Determining where to start 1a. Get partners on board 1b. Review current status of community child health strategy development, planning, and implementation	• Meetings with key persons to exchange information (IMCI and other key programmes, NGOs, partners, other sectors, district and community representatives) • Establish a community IMCI sub-group (if such a group does not already exist) • Sub-group meets to exchange ideas about current activities and agrees upon terms of reference for the sub-group	• Identification of key players in community child health • Overview of recent and current community child health activities and health communication efforts • Identification of entry points and next steps • Formation or strengthening of sub-group	

A. National level planning process for community IMCI (continued....)

Step/Phase	Activities	Outcomes	Comments
2. Understanding the context and building consensus			
2a. Situation analysis at national level	• Sub-group plans situation analysis and adapts IAWG assessment tool, if needed • Sub-group gathers existing data (reports, surveys, evaluations, lessons learned, etc.) • Sub-group interviews key informants at national level and liaises with district coordination committees for information from key informants at district and community level • Sub-group makes site visits	• Description of the national context • Inventory of interventions implemented and lessons learned • Description of available and potential resources	
2b. Share situation analysis with stakeholders	• Organize meeting for sharing results of the situation analysis and discussing next steps (preparatory and/or follow-up meetings may be needed)	• Information exchanged • Agreement on next steps for strategy development	
2c. Review the composition of the sub-group	• Add new members or remove members from the sub-group, as needed	• Sub-group strengthened	
3. Developing national strategy and plan			
3a. Prepare draft national strategy	• Consultations and sub-group meetings to develop and refine draft national strategy and plan	• National strategy (draft) • National plan (draft) • Districts selected for initial support	
3b. Develop national plan (three to five years)	• Hold workshop with representative of stakeholders, regions, districts, NGOs, etc. to share draft national strategy and plan and obtain consensus	• Consensus of stakeholders on national strategy and plan	
3c. Obtain consensus			

B. District and community level planning process for community IMCI

Step/Phase	Activities	Outcomes	Comments
1. Setting the stage for community interventions 1a. Get partners on board 1b. Review current status of community child health interventions	• Find out who is involved in community child health activities in the district, including local and international NGOs, other ministries, women's union, etc. • Invite key players, including representatives of communities, to participate in a group/committee that will coordinate/manage community IMCI in the district (if such a group does not already exist) • Committee meets to exchange ideas about current activities and agrees on terms of reference	• Identification of key players in community child health • Overview of current community child health efforts • Identification of entry points and next steps • Formation or strengthening of coordination committee	The first and second activities could be carried out by district health staff (maybe in collaboration with national IMCI working group).
2. Understanding the context and building consensus 2a. Situation analysis at district and community levels	• Coordination committee plans situation analysis and adapts IAWG assessment tool, if needed • Coordination committee gathers existing information (HIS data, surveys, evaluations, qualitative data reports, lessons learned, etc.) • Coordination committee interviews key informants at district and community levels about their activities and lessons learned • Coordination committee conducts in-depth assessment of key practices and child health needs in selected communities. This might include PRA, ethnographic data collection, and other tools.	• Description of district and community context • Inventory of ongoing interventions and experiences • Lessons learned in child health (and other sectors?) • Description of available and potential resources • Description of current key practices at community and household levels	This step can probably be streamlined by using existing data sources (e.g. KAP survey reports, qualitative data reports, PRA reports, etc.).

REGIONAL FRAMEWORK FOR COMMUNITY IMCI

B. District and community level planning process for community IMCI (continued...)

Step/Phase	Activities	Outcomes	Comments
2b. Share situation analysis results with stakeholders 2c. Review the composition of the coordination committee	• Coordination committee analyses information collected and plans for sharing it • Coordination committee organizes a meeting of stakeholders to share situation analysis results and discuss next steps • Add new members (or remove members) from the coordination committee, as needed	• Information exchanged • Initial agreement on next steps • Communities selected for initial activities • Coordination committee strengthened	Community members should be involved in this meeting. Additional community meetings to discuss the results may be desired.
3. Developing action plans at community level 3a. Obtain participation and involvement of communities 3b. Prioritize family and community practices to address 3c. Choose approaches and activities	• Discuss situation analysis findings • Reach consensus on priority practices to target • Discuss intervention options, types of activities, roles and responsibilities of community members and partners • Develop action plans with community representatives and their partners • Identify resources required and where they will come from • Validate the plans with the wider community • Discuss indicators for monitoring and evaluation	• Community action plans developed • Community level coordination mechanisms, roles and responsibilities, and contributions defined • Detailed input for district level planning obtained	This step could be undertaken by the full coordination committee or by one or more members of the committee depending on the local situation. The community planning could be done through PRA or other participatory planning processes. If funding is needed for community activities (e.g. for training), resources should be identified in advance of community level planning.

B. District and community level planning process for community IMCI (continued...)

Step/Phase	Activities	Outcomes	Comments
4. Developing operational plan at district level 4a. Prepare draft district operational plan (3-5 years) 4b. Obtain consensus	• Coordination committee develops a draft district operational plan using input from the situation analysis and community level planning • Coordination committee holds workshop with stakeholders to obtain consensus on district plan • Based on input from workshop, coordination committee finalizes district operational plan	• District operational plan developed • Consensus of stakeholders on district plan	

NOTES: HIS = HEALTH INFORMATION SYSTEM
IAWG = INTERAGENCY WORKING GROUP ON HOUSEHOLD AND COMMUNITY IMCI
IMCI = INTEGRATED MANAGEMENT OF CHILDHOOD ILLNESS
KAP = KNOWLEDGE, ATTITUDE AND PRACTICE
NGO = NONGOVERNMENTAL ORGANIZATION
PRA = PARTICIPATORY RURAL APPRAISAL

ANNEX 2

INDICATORS FOR IMCI AT HOUSEHOLD LEVEL
(REV 1, JUNE 2001)

Contents

Priority Indicators for IMCI at Household Level

Proposed Supplemental Measures for IMCI at Household Level

Department of Child and Adolescent
Health and Development

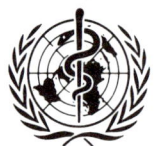

World Health Organization
Geneva
In collaboration with
The Interagency Working Group on IMCI Monitoring and Evaluation
(BASICS, CDC, UNICEF, USAID, WHO)

Topical List of Priority Indicators for IMCI at Household Level

Nutrition

20. Child under 6 months of age is exclusively breast-fed
21. Child aged 6-9 months receives breast milk and complementary feeding
22. Child under 2 years of age is low weight for age

Prevention

23. Child 12-23 months of age is vaccinated against measles before 12 months of age
24. Child sleeps under an insecticide treated net (in malaria risk areas)

Home case management

25. Sick child is offered increased fluids and continued feeding
26. Child with fever receives appropriate antimalarial treatment (in malaria risk areas)

Care seeking

27. Caretaker knows at least two signs for seeking care immediately

Priority Indicators for IMCI at Household Level

(When specified, age groups include children aged exactly the lower number of months up to the end of the upper number of months. As an example, 12-15 months means children aged exactly 12 months up to one day less than 16 months. When age groups are not specified, indicators refer to children up to 5 years of age.)

20. Child under 6 months of age is exclusively breast-fed. Proportion of infants aged less than 4 months who were exclusively breast-fed in the last 24 hours

    Numerator: Number of infants aged less than 4 months (less than 120 days) who were exclusively breast-fed in the last 24 hours.

    Denominator: Number of infants aged less than 4 months (less than 120 days) surveyed.

21. Child aged 6-9 months receives breast milk and complementary feeding. Proportion of infants aged 6-9 months receiving breast milk and complementary foods

    Numerator: Number of infants aged 6-9 months who received breast milk and complementary foods[a] in the last 24 hours.

    Denominator: Number of infants aged 6-9 months surveyed.

22. Child under 2 years of age who is low weight for age (underweight prevalence). Proportion of children who are below -2SD from the median weight for age according to the WHO/National Center for Health Statistics (NCHS) reference population.

    Numerator: Number of children under 2 years of age whose weight is below -2SD from the median weight of the WHO/NCHS reference population for their age.

    Denominator: Number of children under 2 years of age surveyed.

23. Child 12-23 months of age is vaccinated against measles before 12 months of age. Proportion of children aged 12-23 months vaccinated against measles before 12 months of age.

    Numerator: Number of children aged 12-23 months vaccinated against measles before 12 months of age.

    Denominator: Number of children aged 12-23 months surveyed.

---

[a] *Solid and/or semi-solid foods.*

24. Child sleeps under an insecticide treated net (in malaria risk areas). Proportion of children who sleep under insecticide treated[b] nets in malaria risk areas.

   Numerator: Number of children who slept under an insecticide treated net the previous night.

   Denominator: Number of children surveyed.

25. Sick child is offered increased fluids and continued feeding. Proportion of sick children for whom the caretaker offered increased fluids and continued feeding.

   Numerator: Number of children who were reportedly sick in the previous two weeks and for whom the caretaker offered increased fluids and the same amount or more food.

   Denominator: Number of children surveyed who were reportedly sick in the previous two weeks.

26. Child with fever receives appropriate treatment. Proportion of children with fever who received an appropriate antimalarial treatment (in malaria risk areas).

   Numerator: Number of children who were reported to have had fever in the previous two weeks and were treated with a locally recommended antimalarial.

   Denominator: Number of children surveyed who were reported to have had fever in the previous two weeks.

27. Caretaker knows at least two signs for seeking care immediately. Proportion of caretakers who know at least two signs for seeking care immediately.

   Numerator: Number of caretakers of children who know at least two of the following signs for seeking care immediately[c]: child not able to drink or breast-feed, child becomes sicker despite home care, child develops a fever (in malaria risk areas or if child aged less than 2 months), child has fast breathing, child has difficult breathing, child has blood in the stools, child is drinking poorly.

   Denominator: Number of caretakers of children surveyed.

---

[b]*Insecticide treated net include immersion in an insecticide solution and/or regular direct spraying.*

[c]*Local terms to be identified.*

Topical List of Proposed Supplemental Measures for IMCI at Household Level

Nutrition

S19.   Continued breastfeeding rate of children aged 12-15 months

S20.   Complementary feeding frequency

S21.   Stunting prevalence

S22.   Wasting prevalence

S23.   Mean weight for age z-score

S24.   Mean height for age z-score

S25.   Mean weight for height z-score

Prevention

S26.   Diptheria, pertussis and tetanus (DPT) vaccine coverage

S27.   Polio vaccine coverage

S28.   Tuberculosis vaccine coverage

S29.   Vitamin A supplementation

Home case management

S30.   Ownership of mother's card for children under 2 years

Morbidity

S31.   Prevalence of night-blindness

S32.   Period prevalence of history of fever

S33.   Prevalence of malaria parasitemia

S34.   Period prevalence of diarrhoea

S35.   Period prevalence of acute respiratory infections needing assessment

Proposed List of Supplemental Measures for IMCI at Household Level

(When specified, age groups include children aged exactly the lower number of months up to the end of the upper number of months. As an example, 12-15 months means children aged exactly 12 months up to one day less than 16 months. When age groups are not specified, indicators refer to children up to 5 years of age.)

S19. Continued breast-feeding rate of children aged 12-15 months. Proportion of children aged 12-15 months receiving breast milk

    Numerator: Number of children aged 12-15 months who received breast milk in the last 24 hours.

    Denominator: Number of children aged 12-15 months surveyed.

S20. Complementary feeding frequency. Proportion of children aged 1-4 years receiving five or more feeds a day

    Numerator: Number of children aged 12-59 months who received five or more feeds in the last 24 hours.

    Denominator: Number of children aged 12-59 months surveyed.

S21. Stunting prevalence. Proportion of children who are below - 2 SD from the median height for age of the WHO/NCHS reference population.

    Numerator: Number of children whose height (or length) is below - 2 SD from the median height (or length) of the WHO/NCHS reference population for their age.

    Denominator: Number of children measured.

S22. Wasting prevalence. Proportion of children who are below - 2 SD from the median weight for height of the WHO/NCHS reference population.

    Numerator: Number of children whose weight is below - 2 SD from the median weight of the WHO/NCHS reference population for their height (or length).

    Denominator: Number of children weighed and measured.

S23. Mean weight for age z-score. Mean z-score of weight for age according to the WHO/NCHS reference population.

    Definition: Arithmetic mean of weight for age z-score of surveyed children according to WHO/NCHS reference population.

S24. **Mean height for age z-score.** Mean z-score of height for age according to the WHO/NCHS reference population.

Definition: Arithmetic mean of height (or length) for age z-scores of surveyed children according to the WHO/NCHS reference population.

S25. **Mean weight for height z-score.** Mean z-score of weight for height according to the WHO/NCHS reference population.

Definition: Arithmetic mean of weight for height (or length) z-scores of surveyed children according to the WHO/NCHS reference population.

S26. **DPT vaccine coverage.** Proportion of children aged 12-23 months fully immunized against DPT before 12 months of age.

Numerator: Number of children aged 12-23 months who received three doses of DPT vaccine before 12 months of age.

Denominator: Number of children aged 12-23 months surveyed.

S27. **Polio vaccine coverage.** Proportion of children aged 12-23 months fully immunized with oral polio vaccine (OPV) before 12 months of age.

Numerator: Number of children aged 12-23 months who received 3 or more doses of OPV before 12 months of age.

Denominator: Number of children aged 12-23 months surveyed.

S28. **Tuberculosis vaccine coverage.** Proportion of children aged 12-23 months immunized against tuberculosis (BCG vaccine) before 12 months of age.

Numerator: Number of children aged 12-23 months who received a dose of BCG vaccine before 12 months of age.

Denominator: Number of children aged 12-23 months surveyed.

S29. **Vitamin A supplementation.** Proportion of children 6-59 months of age who received a high dose (amount to be defined locally) of vitamin A in the last six months (in countries where there is a vitamin A supplementation policy[d]).

Numerator: Number of children aged 6-59 months who received a recommended dose of vitamin A within the last six months (in countries where there is a vitamin A supplementation policy[d].

Denominator: Number of children aged 6-59 months surveyed.

---

[d] *Some countries may have an upper age limit of less than 59 months.*

S30. Ownership of mother's counseling card for children under 2 years. Proportion of children under 2 years old whose caretaker has a mother's counseling card (in settings where caretakers should receive a mother's counseling card).

    Numerator: Number of children under two years old whose caretaker produces a mother's counseling card.

    Denominator: Number of children under two years old surveyed.

S31. Prevalence of night-blindness. Proportion of children aged 24-59 months who are night-blind (in areas with vitamin A deficiency).

    Numerator: Number of children aged 24-59 months who are reported to be night-blind by their caretaker.

    Denominator: Number of children aged 24-59 months surveyed.

S32. Period prevalence of a history of fever. Proportion of children under five with a report of fever in the two weeks preceding the interview in malaria risk areas.

    Numerator: Number of children for whom the caretaker reports one or more episodes of fever in the previous two-week period.

    Denominator: Number of children surveyed.

S33. Period prevalence of diarrhoea. Proportion of children who had diarrhoea at any time in the two-week period prior to the survey.

    Numerator: Number of children who had diarrhoea at any time in the 2-week period prior to the survey.

    Denominator: Number of children surveyed.

S34. Period prevalence of acute respiratory infections needing assessment. Proportion of children reported to have had fast and/or difficult breathing, with or without cough, in the 2-week period prior to the survey.

    Numerator: Number of children reported to have had fast and/or difficult breathing, with or without cough, at any time during the two-week period prior to the survey.

    Denominator: Number of children surveyed.